Resilient on Purpose

Resilient on Purpose

SHINESE M. COLLINS

Copyright © 2016 by Shinese M. Collins

All rights reserved. Except as permitted under the US Copyright Act of 1976, no part of this publication may be reproduced, distributed, or transmitted in any form or by any means, or stored in a database or retrieval system, without prior written permission of the author.
Shinese Collins, LLC
P.O. Box 15926
Chesapeake, VA 23328

First Edition
ISBN: 9781534679382
ISBN: 1534679383
Library of Congress Control Number: 2016909820
CreateSpace Independent Publishing Platform
North Charleston, South Carolina
This publication is intended to provide inspiration and motivation. It is not intended to treat, diagnose, prevent, or cure any mental health conditions, nor is it intended to replace the advice of a psychologist. The author and publisher specifically disclaim all responsibility for any liability, loss, or risk, personal or otherwise, which is incurred as a consequence of reading or following advice or suggestions in this book.

ACKNOWLEDGMENTS

I thank God for giving me the boldness to share some of my personal experiences. My faith in God has sustained me and carried me through some really tough times.

I also want to thank my husband for being supportive and allowing me to fulfill my dreams. I look forward to many more years together as husband and wife. I am thankful for my pastor and his wife, for their prayers and words of encouragement during these difficult moments.

I am truly grateful for loving friends who have laughed, cried, and prayed with me over the years. Words cannot express how thankful I am for Theresa having shared in this experience with me and contributing the foreword. A special thanks is owed to my daughter for believing in me and always encouraging me.

DEDICATION

I dedicate this book to Hattie and Ernest—may you continue to rest in heaven. You sacrificed so much for me, and I will be eternally grateful for that. I owe both of you so much for teaching me how to get through this thing we call life. Thank you for raising me, teaching me, loving me, making sure I was educated, and for always being there. Thank you for sharing with me the importance of having a relationship with God. I love and miss you both, but I know that you are in my heart. I also know that you are watching over me from heaven.

Love always and forever,
Shinese

CONTENTS

Acknowledgments	v
Foreword	xi
Created to Overcome	1
Desiring a Baby	12
Widowed Overnight	23
Devastated by Dementia	31
Transformation	38
Blessed in Dark Places	45
Forgiveness	55
Strong Women Are Misunderstood	62
Step into Your Excellence	68
About Shinese	77

FOREWORD

Life must be defined; the word alone is full of magnitude. For a moment before you commence reading this inspiring, life-transforming, and impressive literary work by Shinese M. Collins, I want you to think about what life means to you. The power to define is the power to fulfill. Our lives should be lived fulfilled. Unintentionally, one can take life for granted. However, when you walk in the full definition of life while embracing every precious moment, you begin to live in purpose. Your life holds tremendous value. Some of us will never know or understand the influence our lives continue to have in the lives of others. There are people encouraged by your life, your walk, and your smile. While reading *Resilient on Purpose*, you will uncover some similarities between your life and Shinese's as she invites us to peek into her journey. The steps she carried out will certainly serve as an inspiration. We don't have to lean to our own understanding but acknowledge God to direct our paths. It is evident that God instructed Shinese to write this book as well as for you and me to read it. Obedience is better than sacrifice, and I commend you on obedience. Understandably, our obedience to God will continue to yield fruit in our lives. Are you prepared to be blessed? Great! Keep reading…

    A great perspective places you in the room of advantage with doors of peace and windows of innovation. Sometimes, all we need is to look at life from a different perspective. This can be momentous because, with the proper perspective, you will conquer anything. There is a harvest awaiting your arrival, and it is contingent upon your passing this test. Listen, a test not passed will be repeated. As you think back at some of your tests, I know that you have no desire to repeat them. Perspective counts in adversity; it is the currency paid to realize our dreams. Some give up on their assignment, become discouraged, and forfeit realizing their dreams with an improper perspective. Proverbs 24:10 reads, "If you faint in the day of adversity, thy strength is small." Do you see why this book is pivotal to shifting your perspective, building your strength, and reaching your next dimension? There is no better time than now. Beware of distractions while reading this book; your opponent does not want you to win in life. It's a good thing you have laser focus, dominion, and authority. It's winning season, and this year is yours.

Another reason some do not win during the hard times is because of a lack of information or implementation. Knowledge and execution give you a biography of faith. Shinese shares with us how to speak and the steps to enhance our beliefs, which will ultimately help us to move mountains. Those mountains may be death of a loved one, illness, insecurity, unforgiveness, debt, or feeling unworthy. All mountains require the foundational battle plan. There is nothing more rewarding than hearing the specific details from a person who actually repeatedly wins the battles of life. James 1:12 reads, "Blessed is the man who remains steadfast under trials, for when he has stood the test he will receive the crown of life, which God has promised to those who love him."

At times life does not offer a straight path. There are three turns of life; you may perhaps be approaching a storm, driving through a storm, or coming out of one. Trials will come as long as you're living, and they are not designed to make you stronger. Trials are designed to take you out or knock you off course. It is your wisdom-led response to the trials that make you stronger and "resilient on purpose." The title alone is encouragement. I'm thankful that this work goes deeper because we overcome by the word of our testimonies. You must read this book in its entirety... it has your answer. Here is a critical piece to understand: It's better to build in the sunshine than it is to build in the storm. You have the right to know how to build your faith, how to win your trials, and how to realize your dreams.

A miracle is happening in your life at this very moment. You have obtained the book that will give you the solution. Your amazing life and your purpose will be fulfilled in this lifetime. I join with the heart of Shinese M. Collins in extending the blessings of God over your life and proclaiming victory in every area. Thank you, Shinese.

Theresa R. Proctor
Minister, author, and speaker

CREATED TO OVERCOME

The Lord himself goes before you and will be with you; he will never leave you nor forsake you. Do not be afraid; do not be discouraged.

—*Deuteronomy 3:18 NIV*

When a child is born, he or she has the expectation of being loved, wanted, and taken care of. I also believe that everyone is not conditioned to be a parent. Being a parent requires commitment, love, and sacrifice. Often, children are born and naturally taken care of by their birth parents. However, many children are born and abandoned, given up for adoption, neglected, taken in by other family members, or another of many other scenarios.

Many of you who probably remember disco, *Soul Train*, miniskirts, bell-bottoms, and platform shoes were born in the 1970s. Consider a little girl born during a cold winter in New York. Her parents were teenagers and probably not ready to be parents, but now there was a baby with teenage parents living in the projects.

With the help of her parents, my birth mother attempted to take care of me and while completing high school. After graduating, she continued to live with her parents, work, and take care of me.

Eventually, we moved into our own apartment. My guess is that the responsibility of being a single mother and working became overwhelming. My birth mother began to get caught up in the street life. As she started neglecting some of her parental duties, her mother began to notice. Her mother's concern increased, and soon my maternal grandparents stepped in and took on the responsibility of raising me.

The most dysfunctional part of my life as a child was that I often saw my biological parents. I lived in the same building as my biological father until I left the big city to go away to college. My biological mother typically didn't live too far away. I would see her from time to time at some family functions. I believe this interaction imparted feelings of neglect and abandonment in me. I have always wondered why they didn't choose to raise me. As I was growing up, my coping mechanisms were to get lost reading books, to make excuses for my biological parents, or to make up stories to ease the pain of feeling unwanted.

Although I continued to see my biological parents, my grandparents were the constant in my life, and I began to refer to them as my parents instead because their behavior was synonymous with the actions of a mom and dad. It was easier for me to just call them Mom and Poppy. Even with all the love I received, I still couldn't shake the feeling of abandonment by my birth parents. I kept those feelings bottled up inside while growing up. I also experienced the hurt of missed graduations, strained family functions, and broken promises by my biological parents. Meanwhile, my biological parents didn't appear to be impacted by not raising me. For the remainder of this book when I say my mom I am referring to my maternal grandma because ultimately that is who she was to me.

Growing up, I was able to establish some good relationships with my biological father's family. I would go to my paternal grandma's apartment often. I played with the cousins, and my aunts picked up the slack of my biological father. I dealt with the pain of my biological father not acknowledging me in public. I would be standing in the lobby of our building, waiting for the elevator, and if he entered the lobby while I was there he wouldn't even speak to me. This can make a child feel as if he or she had done something wrong, or the parent is ashamed of the child, or that the child is invisible and doesn't matter. Regardless of my poor relationship with my biological father, I was always reminded that he was my father.

Things were similar with my biological mother. Of course, my maternal grandparents picked up the majority of the slack for their daughter. I also had an uncle who lived in the home for many years while I was growing up. I played with cousins, and my aunts and uncles filled in as needed. My biological mother would pop in and out of my life, seemingly with no remorse. She didn't seem to be fazed by how I might be feeling living with her parents. She never asked how I felt about us not having a traditional mother-daughter relationship. She has always claimed the title of mom without putting in the work to be my mom. That is something that I have wrestled with my entire life. Regardless of my strained relationship with my biological mother, I was always reminded that she was my "mother."

No one would ever let me forget where I started. My starting point reminded me of pain, but it was my beginning, and without my biological parents, I would not be here. I also know that there are specific instructions in the Bible on how relationships between parents and children should work. This is one that I always struggled with and, admittedly, still do.

The one thing that I don't think either of my biological parents understood was that I didn't long for material things from them. I just wanted their time and attention. I wanted the truth about why they chose not to raise me. I wanted a sincere apology. I wanted to feel as though I mattered, that I wasn't a mistake or a burden. I wanted more than anything to feel that they wanted me. It is important to learn that putting one's trust in people will bring disappointment, while trusting in God will never disappoint.

Finally, there was always the confusion as to whether to write my biological parents' or grandparents' information on school forms, work applications, and college applications. I even noticed sometimes that family and friends would stumble when asking my how my mom was doing. They would then turn around and say, "You know? Your grandma? Well, she's like your mom." I still couldn't seem to escape that constant reminder.

Both my maternal and paternal grandmothers were strong women of faith. They taught me to pray and to be committed and respectful. Initially, I attended a Methodist church in the neighborhood with my godmother when I was a child. I enjoyed singing in the choir and learning about God. Eventually, I decided to visit the Baptist church where both my grandmothers were members. The worship experience was very different, and at eleven years old, I joined the Baptist church and was baptized.

In church, I learned how to read and study the Bible. I joined the choir and enjoyed how the music ministered to my heart and soul. Building a relationship with God helped me to push through my feelings of neglect. My faith in God and the parents who raised me taught me about love, compassion, and the power of prayer.

I could have very well become a statistic. Even a very little bit of research says that a child who grows up in the projects—or should I say a "bad neighborhood"—is less likely to graduate from high school. According to statistics, these children are more likely to be unemployed, on public assistance, unmarried yet have children of their own. Statistics and those who don't know the power of the Lord expected me to fall prey to street life, become a pregnant teen, and drop out of high school.

The funny thing for me is that I didn't view where I grew up as a bad place. Things may be have worsened now, or perhaps that is just how movies and the media created a picture that is not true. For me, I always felt safe in my neighborhood and at school. As kids, we played outside for hours or until the street light came on. Back when I was a child, we loved playing outside and hated being stuck in the house. We would play in the rain, snow, or cold. Trust me—being raised in the projects when I was a kid was nothing like the movie *New Jack City*.

I always had someone speaking positivity over my life—someone telling me that I could go to college, that I could be anything I wanted to be if I put in the work. I had someone telling me to love and respect myself or no one else would.

If you don't have anyone speaking positivity over your life, then please find some new people to associate with. You can also encourage yourself by reading the Word of God and by telling yourself all of the positive and wonderful things about yourself. Negative self-talk can bring you down. It will make you believe that you are not good enough, or it will have you comparing yourself to others. There is only one you, and what God has for you is for *you*. Don't envy someone else's life because you don't know what it cost them to get that life. If you must compare yourself to someone, then compare yourself to who you want to become.

Identify the fruitful characteristics in that person you want to become, and work on developing your personal spin on those characteristics for you.

When I think back to aunts, uncles, cousins, and staff at the after-school program who were strong, positive role models in my life, my memories remind me to pay it forward. I remember being exposed to art, culture, history, and tons of books. My mom always pushed me to go the extra mile in everything that I did. When participating in church programs, she would work with me in advance to ensure that I was prepared. She would also encourage me to do my best. When it came to academics, she was strict on studying and completing my assignments on time. If I got a ninety on a project or test she would say, "That's good, but next time get a ninety-five."

When it came to applying for college, I applied to both local schools and out-of-state schools. I was accepted to schools in my home state and in two other states. Financially, it made more sense to stay home and attend college, but I made the decision to go to college out of state. My parents supported me in every way that they could while I attended school. They were also the only ones who attended my college graduation.

I was thirsty to find what life existed outside the big city and my neighborhood. I learned at an early age not to be a victim of my circumstances nor to use them as a crutch. My mantra became this verse from Philippians 4:13 NKJV: "I can do all things through Christ that strengthens me." My theory is that life is like a card game. We are all dealt our first hand, but it is how we play our hand and strategically make plays going forward that sets up the end of the game.

My parents drove me to Virginia to my college campus and they dropped me off. In an instant, more or less, I had to learn how to fend for myself. I had to make new friends and learn how to share a room. While the transition was difficult, I was often reminded by my mom that I was not a quitter. She reminded me that with God I would make it through college. Being in a smaller city where things closed early and public transportation was minimal was a big adjustment for a girl from New York. Having to eat dinner very early before the cafeteria closed was also necessary since there were limited food options in walking distance after-hours.

During my first couple of years of college, adjusting to life was challenging. I missed home and life in the big city. I didn't attend church during my first few years of college. The freedom I had living away from home caused me, at times, to go against what I was taught to do. I still listened to my gospel music and read my Bible but just didn't feel the need to attend worship. Then I took a job on campus that was part of the work-study program and helped to pay for my school expenses. One of the ladies in the office that I was working in would talk to me about God and her church. Then one Sunday, she offered to pick me up and take me to her church. During that service, I realized how much I missed attending and being part of worship services.

I began visiting several different churches but ended up back at the one that my work-study boss introduced me to. I felt comfortable there. I enjoyed my worship experience at this church. I didn't attend every Sunday, but I attended when I could. I loved the youth choir. They ministered to my soul.

I have always had a thirst for knowledge. Reading and studying the Bible, as well as being a good student, came naturally to me as a child. Whenever I had a tough decision to make, I would go to my mom, and she would always ask me if I had prayed about it. The more I read the Bible, the more I would continue to have hope that I was created for a purpose.

Reading the Bible and seeing how God provided for the underdog (such as David, Gideon, and Rahab), I knew He would provide for me. I knew God would create a path to elevate my life. I was fortunate enough to have other members of my family and staff from the after-school program as positive role models in my life, to be raised in a home where I saw a strong work ethic, to be taught to take care of myself and my belongings, and to know that education was essential to my future. Education was my prescription to not become a statistic.

I always felt a strong connection to God through music. The words to some of the old hymns are very touching. Some of my favorite songs are by Richard Smallwood. Total Praise always stirs something up inside of me. There is a song out now called Worth by Anthony Brown and Group Therapy. That song is very powerful if you haven't heard it you must find it and listen to it. I know and I believe that God has kept me here in this world for a reason. He has a plan for my life that is exceeding and abundantly above all that I could ever ask for or even image.

Although I had some grants, scholarships, and financial aid, I realized the sacrifice my parents made to put me through college, and this also put added pressure on me to succeed in school. By the grace of God, I graduated, and although I had student loan debt, it wasn't as much as it could have been. Many years after I graduated with my undergraduate degree and before becoming a mother, I applied to graduate school. As a result of the tuition assistance program offered by my employer, I was able to obtain an MBA with minimal personal financial investment. My mom was still there helping me every step of the way. I had a full-time job, but she would still send me a gift toward my textbook expenses. I still continue to attend training classes offered by my company, obtain certifications, read books, learn from mentors, and make use of other ways to further my education.

Let me be clear—my faith didn't erase the hope of my biological mother eventually coming to take care of me. But it did make it easier to deal with all the times that she was not there. My faith taught me that God was always there and would never leave me. Trials and tribulations come, but those situations are ones to learn from to prevent the making of future mistakes. Anything worth having requires one to work for it. No one is going to drop the dream life in one's lap, and winning the lottery is highly unlikely. Erase the mentality that makes those things your hope. Pray and ask God to guide you in all that you do. Apply your plan of action, and God will do the rest.

My faith taught me to be grateful to my maternal grandparents for raising me. It taught me to embrace them as my parents because that is the role they were fulfilling. I also learned to always remember to be respectful to the biological parents who brought me into the world. But, most importantly, I learned not to let the mistakes of my biological parents define my life.

God will see you through any circumstance in your life, no matter how big or small, but you must trust and believe in Him. God hears your cry and will wipe away your tears. God will be your mother and your father. God will be your best friend. God will turn things that were meant to harm you into a blessing. So, as a result, I believe that I was created to overcome. I was created to overcome statistics, abandonment, and the negatives that surrounded my life.

■ ■ ■

Cast all your anxiety on him because he cares for you.

—1 Peter 5:7 NIV

Trust in the LORD with all your heart and lean not on your own understanding; in all your ways submit to him, and he will make your paths straight.

—Proverbs 3:5–6 NIV

The LORD is my light and my salvation—whom shall I fear? The LORD is the stronghold of my life—of whom shall I be afraid?

—Psalm 27:1 NIV

Prayer

Dear God, speak to the broken hearts of all children not raised by their biological parents for whatever reason. God, dry their tears and give them hope. Lord, remove their feelings of neglect and abandonment. Heavenly Father, show them that they don't have to look like what they have been through. Show them that they have been created to overcome. Lord, please stand in the gap of the absent parent, and give these lost children the love they are longing for. Please bless those grandparents, family members, stepparents, foster parents, and any others who have assumed the responsibility of caring for children who are not biologically theirs. These blessings I ask in the name of Jesus. Amen.

What have you been created to overcome?

DESIRING A BABY

Children are a heritage of the Lord, offspring a reward from him. Like arrows in the hands of a warrior are children born in one's youth. Blessed is the man whose quiver is full of them. They will not be put to shame when they contend with their opponents in court.

—*Psalm 127:3–5 NIV*

As a little girl, I dreamed that my future would include my being married with two children, living happily ever after. Well, of course, I didn't anticipate the obstacles that came along to interfere with this dream. I got married, and about nine months into our marriage, we began to try to start our family. Most newlyweds know that family and friends can put a lot of pressure on you in the beginning of your relationship to start a family. People don't realize how insensitive they are being when asking, "So, when are you going to have some kids?" Some people don't want children, some do and are waiting until the time is right for them, and others want children but are unable to conceive. Regardless of the reason, this is really a private issue between a husband and wife that friends and family often invite themselves into.

After six months of trying to conceive, I began to worry that something was wrong. I felt that we were young and healthy, so we should have conceived. Needless to say, I was shocked to find out that the problem was with me. It turned out that I had some medical issues preventing me from becoming pregnant. Devastating news. No one wants to be the problem in not conceiving a child nor does anyone want to have health issues.

The issue was that both of my fallopian tubes were blocked. In order to remove the blockage, I had to have surgery. I prayed to God for a successful surgery. Though this was scary, my desire to be a mom was strong, and I underwent surgery to unblock the tubes. My recovery time was a few weeks. After the surgery, the doctor also put me on hormone medications. That was a horrible experience. I didn't like the side effects of the medicine. The entire situation was very stressful. We followed all of the instructions of the doctor, and we were still unsuccessful conceiving.

During some follow-up visits, doctors discovered another medical issue. This also required surgery, this time outpatient surgery. I again prayed to God for a successful surgery. I was apprehensive, but my desire to be a mom was still strong, so I had this surgery as well. My recovery time was a few days. In the coming months, we still were unsuccessful conceiving a child.

I began to feel like a failure, partially because all of the problems we faced were my issues and also because my husband already had a child from a previous relationship. So as a wife, I felt as though I couldn't fulfill one of my duties and have a child. Well, the mind has a way of playing tricks on you, so I began to feel that I was being punished somehow for my biological parents not raising me. Though the two issues are unrelated, my mind somehow made them one of the reasons why I couldn't have a baby. It also didn't help when people would ask, "When are you going to start a family?" It also seemed that everywhere I looked, friends, coworkers, or family members were expecting babies.

When I shared my feelings of inadequacy with friends, I received various responses. Some responses were that I should enjoy life without children—"At least you don't have to try to find a babysitter." I heard, "Why don't you adopt?" and, "Maybe it wasn't meant to be." Things changed when I shared my feelings with my mom. She asked the most important question: "Have you prayed about it?" My mom also urged me not to give up. She asked, "Where is your faith?"

I began praying through my pain. I asked God to heal my body and bless me with a child. I asked God to help me deal with the news reports when I would constantly see people abandoning or harming babies when I couldn't seem to have one. I even wondered if being unsuccessful conceiving was a sign that I wasn't going to be a good mother. Have you ever heard someone say, "An idle mind is the devil's playground"? Be careful what you speak and be mindful of your thoughts. Thoughts can manifest into beliefs or actions. The job of the devil is to destroy, and he really goes to work when you are down, so block him out of your mind at all times. Many times I thought I was being punished for something I had done in the past and that's why I couldn't conceive. Or I thought that since I wasn't raised by my birth mother maybe I would abandon my child so by not having a child of my own that was preventing history from repeating itself. The more I prayed I began to shift my thoughts and eliminate this negativity.

We went to another follow-up visit with my doctor, and she decided to send me to a specialist. It turned out that this specialist had a high success rate in helping couples conceive either naturally or through in vitro fertilization (IVF). During my examination with the specialist, she discovered that my tubes were blocked again, and she too was recommending surgery. Well, we had heard this story before, and I wasn't sure if I wanted to hear it again.

Feeling like this was my last chance, I agreed to have the surgery. I prayed to God yet again for a successful surgery. This surgery uncovered several issues. It turns out that one of my tubes was severely damaged, and they had to remove it. Just think—if my success rate was poor when I had both of my fallopian tubes, just how much had it diminished with just one tube? We were told that we had about an 8 percent chance of conceiving naturally. The doctor was recommending that we seriously consider IVF.

During the surgery, the doctor also discovered that I had stage-two (of four) endometriosis. The doctor explained it in medical terms, and I did my own research later. I had suffered for about twenty years with severe abdominal pain, migraines, and heavy menstrual cycles that lasted up to nine days, but now I knew the medical term for it. There is no cure for endometriosis, and treatment options include pain relievers, hormone therapy, and surgery. Most of the time, over-the-counter pain relievers didn't remove the pain, instead simply dulling it. After a while, it seemed like my body built up a stronger tolerance for the pain. It still existed, but I was able to deal with it a little better at times. I was very frustrated and confused about why no other doctor had come to this conclusion. Receiving this news made me feel like I had received a knockout punch. I still wanted a child, but I also really wanted to be healthy.

After doing research and reading all the material we received from the specialist, we decided not to invest our money in IVF because it was not a guaranteed option, and it was pretty costly.

We also decided that we needed to keep me healthy. At this point, I was totally discouraged, defeated, and hurt.

During one of my dark moments of sadness about not being able to conceive, I prayed yet again to God to have a baby. Then one day I was reading through *Prayers That Avail Much: Volume Two* by Germaine Copeland of Word Ministries Inc. The prayers in the book were more eloquent than my typical prayers on the topic, but the wording of this prayer still somehow caused a shift in me. I began to change my own prayers after reading the prayer titled, "When Desiring to Have a Baby."

I had prayed for many years for God to grant me a child. Then I shifted my prayer from my desire to have a child to asking God to remove my desire to have a child if that was not in His plan for my life. Once I started praying this prayer, my stress started to disappear. I no longer let my desire to have a baby consume and control me. Having a baby was no longer my main focus. I began to have fun again, and I was able to successfully complete graduate school. It seemed that God gave me peace in the situation.

During my last month of graduate studies, I decided to purchase a new vehicle. I went from a midsize sedan to an SUV. It wasn't a huge SUV, but it was an upgrade in size compared to my midsize sedan. Six months after graduating, I learned that I was pregnant. My vehicle upgrade was right on time. It was certainly much easier to transport a baby, car seat, diaper bag, and stroller in an SUV instead of my midsize sedan. It also seemed safer for me and my daughter being in an SUV vs. a midsize sedan. This was both a happy and a scary time.

Of course I was happy that I was finally pregnant, but I was nervous after my first exam with my doctor. I was considered high-risk because I was thirty-six years old and had experienced some previous medical issues. This meant that I had to go to the doctor more often, and additional tests had to be run on my unborn child. There was also concern for us because my husband was not working at that point, so we didn't know how we could afford an addition to our family.

I had trusted God all these years, and He had done more than I could ever ask for or think of, so I had to go with what I knew. I know that God always has a plan, and while we don't agree with His timing, we have to stand firm on His track record. It is because of God that we wake up every morning. He gives us the activity of our limbs, the ability to work and provide for a family, and the ability to serve others.

I had a healthy pregnancy, and I didn't experience any issues. Everyone was genuinely happy for us once we decided to share the news of our little bundle of joy. Three months after finding out we were having a baby, my husband secured a job. While he had a crazy schedule, we still managed. During my pregnancy, I prayed for my unborn child constantly. I prayed for her health and my health. I prayed that she could hear me when I sang to her and read to her. I prayed that she didn't come into the world too early and that she would be fully developed and healthy when she arrived.

Our daughter was born bright-eyed and healthy. Life as we knew it changed dramatically. I learned a lot about myself while on maternity leave. I wanted to be a mother, but I also wanted a career. I searched long and hard to find a childcare provider for my daughter. I couldn't trust my precious gift from God to just anyone.

Now my prayers shifted to keeping my daughter healthy and giving us the means and ability to take care of her. I prayed that I would become the best mother I could be. I prayed that I would never abandon my daughter. I didn't want her to ever feel how I felt as a result of the choices my biological parents had made.

About four months after the birth of our daughter, my husband was contacted about a contractor position that he had applied for almost a year before. He got the position, and it came with a salary that would definitely help us take care of our daughter. Then, two months after his job improvement, I interviewed for a position that would give me a promotion at work. I had interviewed for similar positions in the past but never landed the job. This time I got the job and received a substantial increase in my annual salary. God is a healer, a provider, and a deliverer. God opens and closes doors that we cannot see.

On my daughter's birthday every year I get emotional. In my time alone, I thank God again for granting my desire and giving me such a precious gift. Being a mom has also taught me a lot about love and sacrifice. I travel a lot for work, but I make every effort to be home for my daughter's school activities, dance recitals, and church programs.

My pastor knew about the challenges we faced with infertility because I had often asked him to pray for me. Based on this knowledge, he connected me with another member of the church who was also having trouble conceiving. I was a little apprehensive, but I asked God to give me the words I needed to be effective in this situation. The pastor introduced us, and I began to share my story with her. I also shared with her the prayers that ministered to me from the Copeland book. I would call her, and I would pray for her often. Then one day, I got a call with the exciting news that she was pregnant. She and her husband now have two healthy little girls. In some small way, I feel that my being transparent with her and sharing my story gave her hope and comfort.

I praise God for the opportunity to be obedient and share my experience with someone else. While this was a very private and difficult time in my life, I had to share what God had done for me. The Bible tells us to be a witness. Matthew 5:16 NIV says, "In the same way, let your light shine before others, so that they may see your good works and give glory to your Father who is in heaven." Often when we are going through things, we think that we are the only ones who are having such experiences. While everyone's situation has some differences, you will also find a lot of similarities. Don't miss an opportunity to minister or witness to someone else.

Now don't get me wrong; I am not saying that God is going to give every woman desiring to have a baby a child. What God has for you is for *you*. What I am saying is to be specific in your prayers. Once you make your requests known to the Lord, you have to wait for Him to answer. It may not always be the answer you are looking for, but it is aligned with the plans He has for your life. Then you must accept and be at peace with God's response to your prayers.

I introduced my daughter to God while she was in my womb. Once she was born, I still read the Bible to her and played my favorite gospel music for her. I continue to expose my daughter to God's Word and talk to her about His love and the importance of obedience. I am honored to say that my daughter made the choice to join church at the age of six, and she has since been baptized. She has her own copies of the Bible, and she leads prayer in the mornings on the way to school. We still enjoy gospel music together.

■ ■ ■

Consider it pure joy, my brothers and sisters, whenever you face trials of many kinds, because you know that the testing of your faith produces perseverance. Let perseverance finish its work so that you may be mature and complete, not lacking anything.

—*James 1:2–4 NIV*

Take delight in the LORD, and he will give you the desires of your heart.

—*Psalm 37:4 NIV*

For everyone who asks receives; the one who seeks finds; and to the one who knocks, the door will be opened.

—*Matthew 7:8 NIV*

Do not be anxious about anything, but in every situation, by prayer and petition, with thanksgiving, present your requests to God.

—*Philippians 4:6 NIV*

For you will be a witness for him to everyone of what you have seen and heard.

—*Acts 22:15 NIV*

Prayer

Dear God, comfort those women desiring to have a baby. I pray that these women seek You in their requests and find comfort in the final outcome. I pray that my story helps someone dealing with a similar situation. I also pray for peace for these women and their families. Lord, I pray for all the unborn children; may they be born into loving families. I pray for those children who are abandoned, abused, and neglected. Please cover them with Your arms of protection. Lord, I ask that every parent seek You for guidance in raising children. Lord, I ask that all children feel loved unconditionally. These blessings I ask in the name of Jesus. Amen.

What have you desired for in your life?

WIDOWED OVERNIGHT

The Lord protects strangers; he supports the fatherless and widow, But He thwarts the way of the wicked.

—*Psalm 146:9 NIV*

We were cruising along in life, doing well in our new positions and raising our daughter.

It was July and hot. I was out of town at my first national convention for my sorority. It was the first time that I had ever left my husband alone to take care of our daughter. She was a little over two years old. During that week, we had a system. My husband would call me every morning once he dropped our daughter off so that I would know that they were OK. Then I would call him every evening to see how their day went.

They seemed to be bonding very well during this time without me. Just a few days before I was scheduled to return home, I made my check-in call for the evening. We had our usual conversation, and I remember asking what he had planned for our upcoming ninth anniversary.

He asked me to send him a picture of me via text. I agreed but got caught up doing things. He called back later and said, "Where is my picture?" I said, "I'm going to send it also reminded him that he was home with several pictures of me. Why do you need a picture?" He nonchalantly said he wasn't feeling good, and we said good night.

The next morning my roommate and I were on our way to breakfast, and once we got to the restaurant, I realized I had left my cell phone at the hotel. We went back to the hotel after breakfast to get my phone. I was surprised to see that I didn't have a missed call from my husband indicating that he had dropped our daughter off. I called our house but got the answering machine. I called his cell phone, and I got voicemail. I also sent him a text message. After about an hour with no response, I tried the house and cell phone again. Then I called his office line and left a message.

Hours went by, and I began to get an uneasy feeling in my stomach. So I called my neighbor and asked her to see if she saw his car or him outside. She said his car was still there, but she hadn't seen him all day. She rang the doorbell but didn't get an answer. I continued to call and leave messages. I called his brother to see if he had heard from him. I called his best friend to see if they had talked. I also called his coworker to see if he had gone to work. His brother hadn't spoken with him, and his coworker said he didn't come into the office.

At this point I was panicking, so I called his best friend again and asked him to go my house and check things out. Well, life as I knew it changed after that phone call. His best friend went to the house and found my husband on the floor—dead, with our daughter sitting next to him. I could not believe what I was hearing. We had just talked the night before. What happened? Was my daughter OK? How soon could I get home?

There was so much to do, but I was not alone. God rallied my sorority sisters around me. Once the word spread, the majority of sorority sisters from my local chapter came to my hotel room. They prayed with me, packed my stuff, and got me a flight out first thing the next morning. My roommate shortened her trip and flew back with me so I wouldn't be alone. I will always be eternally grateful for their displays of compassion during my time of need.

My roommate at the conference called one of my daughter's godmothers to pick her up. I had comfort in knowing that my daughter was in good hands until I could get to her the next day. I called my mom, and she was devastated by the news. She made it to my hometown before I did. I didn't have the heart to break the news to my mother-in-law, so I called my brother-in-law instead. I informed him and asked if he could tell the rest of his family.

All I could do was scream and cry. I couldn't pray using words, but God sent me the help I needed because He knew the desires of my heart. When I arrived at the airport in my hometown, there were about ten people waiting for me—my mom, my daughter's godmothers, and my close friends. God sent angels to watch over me and help carry me through all that needed to be done.

On my anniversary, instead of celebrating, I was planning my husband's funeral. I had never planned a funeral before; it can be overwhelming. To be honest, I didn't even know if he had an insurance policy. The arrangements were finalized, and I decided to have a memorial service in our hometown and have his actual funeral and burial in the town he grew up in.

I decided to have an autopsy done on my husband because other than high blood pressure and high cholesterol, I wasn't aware of any health issues that would have caused him to die so suddenly.

I also didn't know if I needed to look out for any future health issues for my daughter. The autopsy revealed that he had congestive heart failure. Because of my decision to have an autopsy done this delayed the process for receiving the life insurance benefits. For approximately five months God provided for my daughter and I. We were able to maintain the lifestyle we were accustomed to until the payment finally came through from the insurance company.

In the blink of an eye, he was gone. I don't know why God spared me from being at home when this happened. I don't know if he suffered. I don't know if my daughter was in her crib and climbed out and found her unresponsive father. There are so many things that I will never know. What I do know is that I see parts of him in our daughter all the time.

Not only was I a widow overnight—I was also a single mother overnight to a two-year-old. We went through so much to have our daughter, and now her father was dead. Someone once said to me that my daughter arrived when she did so I wouldn't be left alone. I don't know if there is any truth to that, but I do know that having to care for my daughter kept me focused. I know that I had to provide for her more than ever at that point.

You have probably heard people say the only things guaranteed in life are death and taxes. I would add that life is precious. Live it to the fullest, and don't put things off for another day because you may never see that day. Tell people you love them. Spend time with your loved ones. But also take time out for yourself. Women tend to be nurturers by nature, but it's important that we take care of ourselves as well as we take care of others.

I prayed to God for answers after everyone left. I had a lot of time alone with God after my daughter went to sleep. I would be up for hours praying, reading the Bible, and watching Suze Orman's show. An unexpected death will make you get your affairs in order and encourage others to do the same. So if you don't have a life insurance policy outside of one with your employer, please get one. Create an emergency fund with six to nine months of expenses in it. Create and file a will. Be clear on what to do with your children, assets, personal property, and so forth. Complete a living will expressing your last wishes for medical care.

I decided to stay in our home because I knew my neighbors pretty well, and they began to help me a lot. What I couldn't deal with was the fact that our whole life had changed, but everything looked the same. So I began to make changes to the house. I decided to do projects that we talked about but never got around to. Once I made significant changes to the house, it became my and my daughter's home. Dating or getting married again was not on my mind my focus was on taking care of me and my daughter. Besides I had many reservations about dating as a single mother with a young daughter.

Ladies, please be careful if you have children, especially girls. It is not wise to expose your children prematurely to a lot of different men if you have started dating again. You should really get to know the person you are dating, and discuss in depth how he feels about children and raising children from a previous relationship. Gain clarity on his spirituality, beliefs, values, and financial stability. Once you feel comfortable with all of your research, you can introduce your companion to your children in an open setting, not in your home. Consider meeting at a mall, playground, church, and so forth. Introduce your companion and your children, and carefully observe their interactions with one another. Follow your gut! Don't put yourself or your children in a bad situation just because you don't want to be alone. Be specific in your prayers to God for a mate. Wait patiently for God to respond.

God showed me how to adjust to living on one income instead of two. I tithed and remained active in church and in my sorority. My personal network truly rallied around me and became my support system, from cutting grass, to helping to clean out the garage and shed, to offering to babysit. Even as a single mom, I didn't miss a beat. God provided in ways that I couldn't even imagine for me and my daughter.

God turned casual acquaintances into lifelong friends. I truly value the friendships that were birthed out of this tragedy. These individuals saw me at my worst and still wanted to be my friend. In the same way, God sees us at our worst and can still find the best in us. My relationship with God became even stronger.

The most important thing I can share about this experience is the importance of not giving up on love. Keep your heart open. If it is in God's will, He will send you another mate. You can have another chance at marriage and building a family. The key is that you must be open and receptive. Also, don't get caught up comparing a new mate to your old mate. We are all different and not created to be exactly the same. Get to know your new companion, and identify what draws you to him, what you love about him, and why you want to spend the remainder of your life with him.

■ ■ ■

The righteous cry out, and the Lord hears, and delivers them from all their troubles. The Lord is near the brokenhearted; He saves those crushed in spirit.

—Psalm 34:17–18 NIV

Peace I leave with you. My peace I give to you. I do not give to you as the world gives. Your heart must not be troubled or fearful.

—*John 14:27 NIV*

Stay alert, stand firm in the faith, show courage, be strong.

—*1 Corinthians 16:13 NET*

Prayer

Dear God, please continue to comfort and watch over widows. Give them peace, and help them to know they are not alone. Remind them not to take life for granted but live it to the fullest. May they feel love from their families and friends. May they hold on to memories of good times shared with their spouses. These blessings I ask in the name of Jesus. Amen.

Have you experienced an unexpected loss, and how does that make you feel?

DEVASTATED BY DEMENTIA

You will keep in perfect peace all who trust in you, all whose thoughts are fixed on you!

—Isaiah 26:3 NLT

I was raised by a faithful, fiery, and strong black woman. She was very active. She worked, traveled, and was very active in her church. When I say active in church, I mean she served as the president of the adult usher board for twenty years. She was also the chairperson of the trustee board for a number of years. She attended Sunday school and loved to sing and read her Bible.

About eight months after my husband passed away, I was home visiting for Easter with my daughter, and my poppy passed away early on Easter Sunday morning. He was eighty-three years old, and he and my mom had been married for more than fifty years. Here I was, less than a year after my husband's death, planning another funeral. For the next few years I tried to persuade my mom to move to Virginia to be closer to me and my daughter. Yet it seemed like my mom took Poppy's death harder than she wanted us to know.

I moved away from home when I was seventeen years old to attend college, and I never moved back. When my mom would visit, we always had a busy schedule. We would try new restaurants and shop. She would help me decorate my house. My friends would come by to visit her, and she treated everyone like they were family. Once my daughter was born, she would visit quarterly to see her granddaughter and to help me out. She would attend worship with me, and she got to know all my friends well. Additionally, my mom and I talked on the phone several times a day.

My mom was known for her style and her skills in the kitchen. Oh, how she cooked some meals that I will always remember. In fact, last year I found myself longing for some of those meals, and I would call her for the recipes. She would guide me through cooking via telephone. My mom was always well known for her beautiful hair. As far back as I could remember, she faithfully got her hair done every two weeks. She never had a strand out of place. Appearance was very important to my mom; she always expected one's clothes to be neat, clean, and ironed. One's hair and nails should always be presentable.

I remarried about three years after my husband's untimely death. These were truly happy times in my life. I felt like my daughter and I had a second chance and a whole family unit. My husband and I purchased a new home, and we started our new life together. Our new family included me, my daughter, my husband, and our dog. All I could see was a happy future ahead with my new husband and family.

Then a few months after our honeymoon and after we had moved into our new home, I began to notice that my mom was repeating herself a lot and becoming very forgetful. I contacted her doctor and shared my observations and concerns. My mother was tested, and the diagnosis was dementia.

It started out with my mom being emotional and frustrated by her memory loss. She would remember things that happened more than twenty years ago but couldn't remember something that had just happened that morning. At times, she would just burst out into tears and say, "I'm losing my mind." I tried my best to comfort her. Sometimes it worked, and sometimes she would just hang up on me.

My mom became fearful, which was tough for me to comprehend because she had always been such a strong woman. I didn't think she was afraid of anything. She confided in me that she would get confused when she was outside, and she was afraid she would get lost. She started to miss paying some of her bills, or she would pay some of them twice in one month. We talked about her struggle, and I took over handling all of her finances. I made sure her bills were paid on time. I would ensure there was money in an account locally so that she could have groceries and other necessities.

Then Mom just stopped going outside, period—very odd for a woman who would go out almost daily to take a walk and get some fresh air. Mom stopped going to get her hair and nails done, which was something that she used to be so meticulous about. She eventually stopped going to church, though she still had her mind fixed on the Lord. Regardless of what kind of day she was having, she always had a word from or for the Lord.

During the last few years when she would visit, she didn't want to go anywhere or do anything. All she would do was eat, sleep, and spend time with my daughter. She would stay in her pajamas all day long, which typically was not acceptable by her standards. I witnessed my mom start to give up on her life. This was tough, so I began learning more about dementia and noticing different stages and symptoms that she was going through.

I began researching assisted living facilities in my area and discussed the possibility of my mom moving near me so that I could care for her better. She would at least talk about it, but she made it clear that she didn't want to live with me, and I knew she couldn't live alone. All of the facilities that specialized in dementia care were costly, and then I tried to find additional funds that could help pay for that care. I was unsuccessful, stressed, and frustrated.

Speaking as the family member of someone with dementia, it is a difficult disease to deal with. At times, I felt like I no longer knew my mom. Or I felt like I was grieving for her although she was still alive; she was just not the woman I always knew. I cherished our phone calls when she was having a good day. Because of her dementia, my vibrant mother became a recluse. She would go through crying spells or at times become very agitated and angry. Dementia is a horrible disease that impacts the whole family.

One night, my mom fell in her apartment on the way to go to bed. She had a fractured hip as a result of the fall. Her only chance to walk again was to have surgery. We consented to the surgery. During pre-op, the doctors discovered that she had major blockage in her arteries. In order to do the hip surgery, they had to insert a stent to open the blockage. Both surgeries were successful.

However, after the surgeries, her dementia seemed to have progressed. She seemed to be easily aggravated. Sometimes it was hard to follow her conversations. She was confused easier than before, and she cried a lot more. My mom's health continued to deteriorate. This put a lot of stress on me, as I was the person responsible for either carrying out her wishes or making decisions about her care.

I spent the last five months of her life talking to doctors, nurses, social workers, and so forth. Making health care decisions, researching medical terms, and asking questions about caring for a loved one can really drain you. If you happen to be in this situation, please remember to take time to care for yourself. During all of this, my mom may not have known what day it was, but she always had a word from or for the Lord. I truly admired her faith.

My prayers initially were for her to get better and for me to move her near me once the doctors confirmed that she could not be permitted to travel. As I had to make decisions for her final care, I began to pray for comfort and peace for both of us. Of course I wanted my mom to be healed and for us to have more time together. But I also didn't want to be selfish. I had to pray that God's will would be done and that I would find comfort and peace in the decisions I had to make on my mom's behalf.

At times, I felt like the weight of the world was on my shoulders. I was overwhelmed by all the decisions I needed to make and by the possibility of losing my mom. I found comfort in expressing my feelings to my closest friends and by talking to God. I know that not all sickness leads to death. I also know that whether one loses someone unexpectedly or expectedly it doesn't make it any easier to deal with. Cherish your time with your loved ones. Don't take those moments for granted. Make sure that you discuss final wishes with your loved ones and get that information in writing—it does help.

■ ■ ■

And be not conformed to this world: but be ye transformed by the renewing of your mind, that ye may prove what [is] that good, and acceptable, and perfect, will of God.

—*Romans 12:2 KJV*

Finally, brethren, whatsoever things are true, whatsoever things [are] honest, whatsoever things [are] just, whatsoever things [are] pure, whatsoever things [are] lovely, whatsoever things [are] of good report; if [there be] any virtue, and if [there be] any praise, think on these things.

—*Philippians 4:8 KJV*

Prayer

Dear Heavenly Father, I pray for a cure for dementia, cancer, and other terminal illnesses. I pray for comfort for the patients and their families. I pray that there is no long suffering. Lord, if it is in Your will to send healing, please send it down. Dear God, I pray for guidance for the caregivers and decision makers. These blessings I ask in the name of Jesus. Amen.

Has your family been impacted by dementia?

TRANSFORMATION

Then Jesus declared, "I am the bread of life. Whoever comes to me will never go hungry, and whoever believes in me will never be thirsty.

—*John 6:35 NIV*

You hear about companies downsizing and restructuring all the time. The new buzzwords are "departmental and organizational transformation." You may even see it happen in other departments but not in yours. When it hits your department and directly impacts you, things become real.

One day, I received the announcement that our department would be undergoing transformation. This means that in the new organizational structure, there was not a position for everyone.

Everyone had to apply for positions that they were qualified for and go through the normal interview process. For the first time in my career, I saw a severance package. The company made the decision to share all of our options with us, with a deadline either to be selected for a new role in the company or to accept the package.

After getting over the initial shock, I took advantage of all the resources offered to us. I updated my résumé and began practicing my interviewing skills. I shared my résumé with my mentors for feedback. I inquired about skills that I thought I might be lacking and sought ways to enhance them. I conducted mock interviews for coworkers in other departments and began to read more about leadership skills.

This process gave me yet another reminder of how often we take things for granted. I had been employed with the same company for eighteen years and never thought that I would be in this situation. It is important to update your résumé, at minimum, once a year. Stay active in networking—don't just reach out to people when you need them, but stay connected. Continuously obtain new skills and enhance existing skills. Track your successes, and articulate them to your board of directors.

I witnessed fear and panic among my coworkers. I often had people make the comment that I had nothing to worry about because of my tenure with the company. I know for a fact that tenure doesn't save one's job. I also know that I had to put my trust in God and put in the work to prepare to go through the transformation process. Although my department was going through this transformation process, we still had our current job responsibilities to fulfill. I continued to perform on my job and volunteered for projects. I helped coworkers when I could with the process.

I learned patience and listened to God during this time. Sometimes updates were not provided in a timely manner, but I didn't panic—I trusted that all things would work out for the good. I looked through my network and shared my current situation with those whom I could trust so that, in the event that I needed to find another job outside the company, I had already started the connection.

I prayed for clear direction and clarity in what jobs to post for in the new organization. I prayed for a calm mind and a courageous spirit. I prayed that all impacted employees would secure employment within or outside the company. I also prayed for the right words to say to my coworkers when they expressed concern over the situation or asked for my advice. Someone is always watching how one reacts to situations, especially when one is a Christian. I prayed that the Jesus in me would shine through.

I could have become consumed with worry over the potential loss of my job after eighteen years. I could have become angry and made premature decisions such as finding permanent employment outside the company. Instead, I made the decision to continue showing up daily and performing my duties to the best of my abilities. I didn't focus on the "would have" but on the here and now.

Going through this transformation at work it reminded me that it is important to live a life that is pleasing to God. If you are a Christian you shouldn't have to tell someone that you are a Christian they should know it by your actions. Now I am not saying that you shouldn't tell people that you are a Christian. What I am saying is your actions and your words should be in sync. If you have faith it should be evident in how you handle situations. As I get older and encounter various obstacles or set-backs in my life I have noticed that my faith does not waiver. My Faith in God (FIG) grows stronger through it all.

My husband was very supportive through the process of my company's transformation. He prayed for me and kept me focused. There is comfort and power in having a spouse who prays for you. With his support and my faith in God, we made it through this test. I was finally offered a position, which turned out to be a promotion.

God continues to grant me favors. It is not because I deserve it. It is because He is a merciful God, and I fully realize to whom much is given, much is required. I praised God in advance and during the announcement of my new position with the company.

Then one day an opportunity presented itself to me three times within one week. While checking my social media account on three separate occasions, I saw the business in a box birthday special appear in my news feed. I inquired about it, and I prayed about it, and during the transformation process I made the decision to learn entrepreneurial skills. I invested in a jewelry business. I purchased a business in a box. I never envisioned myself as a salesperson. However, I went through the online training modules, received my business in a box, and launched my business.

I announced to a small group of people about my business venture and invited them to my launch party. Ten guests attended my launch party. We played games, had refreshments, and tried on fabulous jewelry. Everyone who attended the party made a purchase and a few who were not able to attend made a purchase as well. After my launch party, I totaled up my sales and discovered that I made about 55 percent of my initial investment in the business back during that one event. The best part is that I had a great time doing it.

Of course, the extra money from my business will help to take family vacations and improve our financial portfolio. Our CEO, who is an ordained evangelist, mentors us weekly. She prays for us and with us. She practices tough love with us and teaches us lifelong lessons in business. The business skills that I have learned can be applied to my business and in my corporate job as well. I learned team-building skills that are applicable to my business, to board positions that I hold, and in my corporate job. I have also been able to elevate my relationship-building skills. I also acquired entrepreneurial skills which include how to market a small business, filing taxes for a small business, establishing separate accounts and handling accounts receivables for a small business.

I thought that I was investing in this business to help enhance my financial resources for my family. Unexpectedly, it turned out to be more than that. I have learned so much about myself as a result of this business. I discovered a lot of things that I needed to work on personally in order to grow as a person. This business took my confidence to a level that I didn't know existed. This investment has made me search my soul and dig up my dreams. I have been able to identify the things that I am really passionate about, and I am working on making those dreams my reality.

Through this business investment, I have discovered that I have so much more to offer to the world. This investment in myself has pushed me to share my story with the world. As a result of this small investment, I have not only become a small business owner, but I have found my voice that was buried so deep inside when I was afraid to speak out. I have been able to hear God's voice more clearly now that I have started tearing down walls in my life so that I could grow.

The end result of this time was that my department was transformed and so was I. A change has come over me. I am enjoying getting to know the "me" who was buried so deep within. God is a provider. You must listen for His instructions. You must believe in God and in yourself. Do you have a dream that you have not gone after? It's time to do an assessment of your life. Make sure that what you are doing is something that you are passionate about and find rewarding. Remember, you are never too old to set another goal or to dream a new dream. I love this quote from Joel Osteen: "Start thinking bigger, praying bigger, expecting bigger. God wants to take you where you've never been."

■ ■ ■

Therefore, do not be anxious, saying, "What shall we eat?" or "What shall we drink?" or "What shall we wear?" For the Gentiles seek after all these things, and your heavenly Father knows that you need them all.

—Matthew 6:31–32 ESV

And my God will supply every need of yours according to his riches in glory in Christ Jesus.

—Philippians 4:19 ESV

And without faith it is impossible to please him, for whoever would draw near to God must believe that he exists and that he rewards those who seek him.

—Hebrews 11:6 ESV

Prayer

Dear Lord, I pray for those who have lost their jobs. I pray that they keep the faith and seek Your guidance to find employment. I also pray for those who are employed, that they make wise decisions and show gratitude for having a job. I pray that the employed don't take anything for granted and look to build relationships that will help them in present and future endeavors. I pray that they practice good stewardship principles and never forget those less fortunate. These blessings I ask in the name of Jesus. Amen.

Are you struggling with job loss?

BLESSED IN DARK PLACES

We are confident, I say, and would prefer to be away from the body and at home with the Lord.

—*2 Corinthians 5:8 NIV*

I am no stranger to death. Unfortunately, I've had family and friends pass away throughout my life. I have even had to plan several funerals. But there is no pain as crushing as the pain you feel when you bury you mother. As I mentioned before, my mom had dementia, and one day she fell. She had a few surgeries, and her recovery did not go well. Due to the dementia, rehab was very challenging.

She began becoming more withdrawn, and she stopped eating. Any research on dementia points out that this is typical. As a result of not eating, she was too weak to participate in physical therapy. She began to lose a dramatic amount of weight. Her blood pressure would drop extremely low at times, and the nursing home staff would contact me to discuss options for treatment.

After sending my mom to the emergency room a few times, she told me that she didn't want to go back to the hospital anymore. There came a time when her health was deteriorating, and the doctors had a conversation with me to discuss palliative care if my mom's condition worsened. Although she had many things outlined in legal documents, it was still very difficult to talk about what could be the final days of my mom's life.

This was not an episode of a TV show. This was real life, and I had to make the call on whether or not to do CPR, insert a breathing tube, and so forth. I applaud the doctor for his patience and the time he took to explain all of our options. Nonetheless, it didn't make the pressure of stating my decision out loud any easier. I prayed for comfort for my mom and for guidance from God in the decisions.

Two months later, my mom was still here. She actually seemed to be improving. Then, we took three steps backward, and she was back to not eating again, and her blood pressure was dangerously low. Then she stopped responding to the staff. I was informed that my mom was transitioning, and it was only a matter of time. The last thing I said to my mom is, "I love you." She didn't respond, but I believe she heard me.

Finally, I received the dreaded call that my mom went home to be with the Lord. I was in shock and just felt overwhelmed. I dreaded having to inform my daughter that her Nana was now in heaven. They had been very close. They would read books, sing, and watch TV together, all via telephone. Every time I spoke to my mom, her first question to me was, "How are my girls doing?" My typical response was that we were fine, and she would always say, "If ya'll are all right, then I am OK."

After my mom's death, I was devastated but immediately took on the mindset to handle business affairs. I had a pep talk with myself and told myself that now was not the time to fall apart. Now was the time to keep my head straight, handle the funeral arrangements, and notify any remaining family and friends of her passing. Finally, I made arrangements to get me and my family to the big city so we could attend my mom's funeral. I followed my mom's wishes to the best of my ability when planning her funeral. Although I shed some tears, I knew that the true pain of my loss had not surfaced.

When I walked into my mom's apartment, I felt extremely sad. There were so many memories of my growing up there. It didn't feel like home. It felt like I was a stranger in the place where I grew up. I handled the business I needed to handle and quickly went back to the hotel with my family. During her funeral, I saw some people I hadn't seen in years, and it was a reminder of how loved my mom was. She made an impact on so many lives. The service was very nice. Once it was over, all I wanted to do was go home.

I felt like I didn't belong in the big city anymore now that my mom was gone. We had so many memories there. We experienced joy and pain there. My heart was broken and ached for just one more hug from my mom. I just wanted to hear her voice again or her infectious laugh. However, I was glad to know that she was no longer suffering. I know that she is with the Lord and has no more pain, her mind is renewed, and she is singing in the angelic choir. When I close my eyes, I still see her face. I sometimes smell her perfume when I walk throughout my house. I often still hear her words of encouragement and wisdom as a whisper in my ear when I am having a quiet moment.

She was my mother/grandmother, friend, prayer partner, counselor, comforter, and cheerleader. She practiced tough love with me, and while I didn't understand it when I was growing up, I appreciated it as an adult. She taught me how to run a household, handle business affairs, and be respectful. She insisted that I always show gratitude when someone was kind to me with a gift. I always had to handwrite a thank-you note. She taught me to study the Word of God, to pray, and to give thanks. But now she is gone after eighty-two years on this earth.

The irony of the passing of my mom is that my biological mom is still living. We are basically estranged. We don't really know each other in the traditional sense of a mother and daughter. I have not closed the door on this relationship, but I will admit that it has been a challenge to leave it open.

A few hours before my family and I left the big city, I received a phone call that my paternal grandma passed away. This could not be happening so soon, all at once. I still had not come to terms with the passing of my mom. So many more emotions came rushing upon me. Would I be able to return to the same church where my mom was buried to pay my final respects to my grandma? I couldn't believe that I was feeling claustrophobic in such a big city.

My paternal grandmother had also suffered with dementia and other health issues. She had raised ten children, including my biological father. Although he and I didn't have a relationship, I did have one with his mom. As a child, I would visit her apartment, and we would spend time together, or my cousins and aunts would be there, and we would all spend time together. She was truly the matriarch of the family after my grandfather passed away when I was around eleven or twelve years old.

She taught me how to respect myself, how to be strong, and how to take care of a family. I was always guaranteed to get a good laugh whenever I visited or talked to grandma on the phone. When I left the big city to go away to college, I didn't keep in touch as much as I should have, but we would always connect when I returned to the city during my school breaks. My grandma was a strong woman, full of life and love. She had strong faith and was very active in our church before she became ill. She will be missed but will always live in my heart.

I cried so much the day of my grandma's funeral (incidentally, my maternal grandfather's birthday); I thought that the grieving process had to have begun. But it seems that I had not even scratched the surface. Then I had to go out of town on a business trip. When I got back to my room that first night, I went to call my mom, and it hit me that she was gone. That was a sick feeling because we spoke so often and especially when I was traveling.

I thought that I would finally start dealing with the loss of my mom and my grandma. I buried myself in work and other activities because I was afraid to face my feelings. I reminded myself that they were no longer suffering, and they were rejoicing in heaven. That didn't make it any easier to accept the truth.

By this time, my uncle had been struggling with his health for over a year. He fell and fractured his leg in multiple places and had five surgeries on that one leg. He was bedridden for at least six months. The man who was once a basketball star now required a wheelchair to get around.

We would trade text messages; he would write me letters; and we talked via phone from time to time. I would also send him care packages. It was comforting to see my uncle reference specific Bible verses and talk about God during our conversations though he didn't believe in attending church.

Then, nineteen days after my grandma's funeral, I received a phone call that my uncle had passed away. We were twelve years apart in age, but he was a very integral part of my life growing up. He was kind of like the older brother I never really had. He scared away my boyfriends when I was a teenager. He helped me with my homework, and he taught me about sports and music. He loved to play basketball, and he was pretty good. He played in high school and some in college. I would often watch him play in the neighborhood.

He had not put any of his final wishes in writing nor had he discussed them with me. Now that he was gone, I needed to make the arrangements. My uncle wasn't married and didn't have any children. I truly struggled making the arrangements for his service because I didn't know his religious preferences. Despite all of my agonizing, his memorial service was very nice and well-attended.

I plead with you to get your affairs in order. Make your final wishes known verbally and in writing. Don't leave the burden of making these decisions on your loved ones. Experiencing three deaths so close in time and in my immediate family was a big blow. It is difficult to process, and it can take your breath away. My head was spinning, and I mostly felt numb. I really looked to the Word of God to find direction and comfort.

After suppressing my feelings in order to plan services and handle personal business for my family members, I prolonged the grieving process. Because of that, there are so many feelings bottled up inside. I have people constantly telling me that they are praying for me. I truly appreciate that, but please know that I am still praying for myself. I also know that it is important to go through the grieving process and talk about my feelings. I have been journaling, and that is helping. I continue to pray, and I must admit that when I finally started to feel the back-to-back losses of my loved ones, it hit like a ton of bricks. I would have these crying episodes when I just couldn't stop. I even felt like I couldn't breathe at times.

Talking about my feelings and meditating on God's word have truly been helpful. I know that God still has his hands of protection and love around me. I know that God will dry my tears and comfort me. I believe that my mom, grandma, and uncle are all in a better place and are no longer suffering in their earthly bodies. They all died in approximately a thirty day period of time. While I feel a void from all these losses, I believe that God still has great things in store for me.

I know that my loved ones would want me to move on with my life. I know that my daughter and my husband need me to be present and active in their lives. I know that the pain will fade, yet the memories will always remain in my heart. I know that, with help from God, I will recover from this grief storm and be victorious. Remember that your loved ones may be gone, but you are still alive. So live the rest of your life to the fullest. I still hear my mom's voice at times. I hear her encouraging me to pursue my dreams. I hear her telling me that I'm going to make it and to hold to God's unchanging hands.

People see me, and they say, "You are so strong after all that you have been through." I don't feel strong. I know that in my weakness God gives me strength to move forward. I've also had people say that they don't know what to say to me. Well, my thoughts typically are that I don't know what to say to them either. So why not talk about something else besides grief or loss?

During one of my quiet moments, I realized that I was no longer juggling work, being a mom and a wife, and making long-term care decisions for my mom, handling her financial affairs, and checking on and providing for my uncle. While it hurt deeply to lose my loved ones, the end result was that I had a lot more time available. This made me see that while I am grieving the loss of my loved ones, God has given me freedom to focus on me for the first time in a long time. God has blessed me to strengthen my relationship with Him. He is giving me peace and clarity in some situations where I didn't have any before. He is tearing down strongholds from my life. I am rejoicing in the glory of the Lord. God is birthing new ideas and waking up old dreams in my life. I know this is true because you are reading this book, which came about through my conversations with God. God is stirring up gifts inside me that I have kept buried for far too long.

So I say to you, do not be consumed by your grief, but do go through the grieving process. Stay connected to God, and He will carry you through. Find peace in His Word, and remember what God has already done for you in your life. Hold to God's unchanging hands, and press forward. Find a grief counselor or group where you can share and understand your feelings. Give yourself permission to feel whatever you feel, whether it's sadness, anger, or loneliness. You must feel and move on; don't get stuck.

■ ■ ■

> *For everything there is a season, and a time for every matter under heaven: a time to be born, and a time to die; a time to plant, and a time to pluck up what is planted; a time to kill, and a time to heal; a time to break down, and a time to build up; a time to weep, and a time to laugh; a time to mourn, and a time to dance.*
>
> —*Ecclesiastes 3:1–4 ESV*

> *Do not let your hearts be troubled. You believe in God; believe also in me. My Father's house has many rooms; if that were not so, would I have told you that I am going there to prepare a place for you?*
>
> —*John 14:1–2 NIV*

Brothers, I do not consider that I have made it my own. But one thing I do: forgetting what lies behind and straining forward to what lies ahead, I press on toward the goal for the prize of the upward call of God in Christ Jesus.

—Philippians 3:13–14 ESV

He will wipe every tear from their eyes. There will be no more death or mourning or crying or pain, for the old order of things has passed away.

—Revelation 21:4 NIV

Prayer

Dear Heavenly Father, I pray for all families who have experienced the death of a loved one. I pray for those individuals who have to make the final arrangements for their loved ones. May they seek You in all the decisions they need to make, and may they find peace in You. Lord, wrap Your loving arms around these grieving individuals. Make it known that they are not alone and that You are with them always. Lord, only You can heal our hearts, minds, and bodies. Thank you, God, for being an omnipresent and a forgiving God. These blessings I ask in the name of Jesus. Amen.

What blessings have you received in your dark moments?

FORGIVENESS

In him we have redemption through his blood, the forgiveness of our trespasses, according to the riches of his grace, which he lavished upon us, in all wisdom and insight making known to us the mystery of his will, according to his purpose, which he set forth in Christ as a plan for the fullness of time, to unite all things in him, things in heaven and things on earth.

—Ephesians 1:7–10 ESV

Most often when we think of forgiveness, we think of what it will do for the other person. While it is good for the person who wronged us, it's really best for the person who was wronged. I know firsthand how damaging not forgiving someone is. Holding a grudge or being unforgiving hardens your heart. Failure to forgive is like a disease because it can infect your physical, mental, and emotional being. It can consume your mind, cause unnecessary stress, and make you do childish things.

Think about how many adults you know who go out of their way not to speak to someone with whom they have an unresolved issue. How often is someone's lack of forgiveness of another the topic of gossip? How often does it sever relationships or create barriers in their communication? Ultimately, not forgiving someone can be a major drain on one's energy level.

So, as a Christian, asking for forgiveness is usually part of our prayers. How can you ask God to forgive you when you won't forgive one of His children? How can we teach our children about forgiveness when we don't practice what we teach? God gave us the ultimate display of forgiveness by letting His son Jesus die on the cross to erase our sins.

Lack of forgiveness can impact other relationships in a person's life. Remember that someone is always watching how you react or handle situations. When people know you are unforgiving toward someone, that knowledge can damage their perception of your character. It may cause you to be perceived as a hypocrite. It can send mixed messages to your children. It could even impact how you are perceived at work.

Remember that God knows your thoughts even when you don't verbally communicate that you are not forgiving someone. You may keep your mouth closed, but even your body language can send messages about how you feel about a person or situation. By not forgiving someone, you are giving them control over a portion of your life.

I have had to pray for forgiveness many times. I have also had to forgive myself and others. I had to forgive my biological parents for not raising me. I had to forgive myself for the anger and disappointment I felt when my biological parents didn't acknowledge my birthday or other special events in my life. I had to forgive myself for letting fear or doubt consume me at times and not stepping into the greatness that is inside of me. I had to forgive myself for feeling that it was my fault that my mother's health deteriorated because I didn't make her move. I had to forgive myself for questioning why God took my mom, grandma, and uncle from me in such a short period of time, for the selfishness of not wanting them to leave me though they were all suffering from health issues.

Another part of forgiveness is forgiving oneself. Most of the time, I am harder on myself than I am on others. I can be my own worst enemy. Get out of your own way and forgive yourself. We all make mistakes. We sometimes have poor judgment or make bad decisions. Before we can mend relationships with others, we have to improve our personal perceptions of ourselves.

Once you make the decision to forgive—when and if it is appropriate—you should tell the person that you forgive him or her. If you have the opportunity to speak with the person one-on-one in a private setting that is the perfect opportunity to express your forgiveness. This step will help both of you move on. If you are not able to talk in person, consider writing a letter. By writing the letter it allows you to release all the feelings you have about the situation or the person. Informing someone of your forgiveness is important because they may not realize that they have offended or hurt you. You may even discover that the entire situation was a big misunderstanding by both of you. In life, it's best to assume positive intent from everyone. Expect that people will not intentionally hurt you. Having those conversations and forgiving others can relieve stress, open doors, and, above all, is pleasing to God.

During a sermon one Sunday, the pastor was preaching about forgiveness. I went home that day and called my biological mom and told her that I forgave her. I let her know that we could still have a relationship but that it would take work and commitment from both of us. Several times since then we have had some good moments, but then something came up and we stopped communicating again.

I knew and shared my feelings about my biological mom, but I realized that I had never told my biological father how I felt. This became clear to me one day when I was watching a movie in which the dad was a police officer and his young daughter died. The dad really struggled as he thought of all the things he would never get to do and experience with his daughter. It was very emotional. That is when I realized that I had never taken the chance to tell my biological father how I felt. A few days later, I sat down and wrote him a long letter pouring out my feelings. Several months after that, he acknowledged receipt of my letter and said he planned to respond. It has been about four years, and I have not received a response. However, I do have peace because I was able to let him know how I truly felt and what an impact he had on my life by not being there. I also extended the invitation for us to get to know each other and build a relationship, but nothing has happened since I opened that door. But, I am in a better place because I forgave him and let him know that I did.

God's Word is clear on how to handle forgiveness. When in doubt, always pray to God for direction. Seek God for the specific words to communicate your forgiveness. Be genuine when you are forgiving someone and when you are asking for forgiveness. I understand that forgiveness doesn't mean that we forget what had been done to us. But once we forgive, we should feel shackles being released. That is when your prayers can change to ask God to remove the pain or the memory of the act. You can pray to God to replace that pain with love. Consider this quote by Gary Zukav author of *The Seat of the Soul*: "An authentically powered person lives in love. Love is the energy of the soul. Love is what heals the personality. There is nothing that can't be healed by love. There is nothing but love."

Pray that God will help you forgive yourself for the things that are keeping you stuck in your past. Pray for healing of those acts, and watch the shackles be removed. Break every chain with the power of God, forgiveness, and love. It's time to love yourself; start by being diligent in forgiving. We all have flaws. We are all a work in progress. But know that God is not finished with you yet. So keep on improving yourself. Open your heart and mind to the endless possibilities God has in store for your life. God already made the first move. Now it's your turn.

■ ■ ■

For if you forgive men when they sin against you, your heavenly Father will also forgive you. But if you do not forgive men their sins, your Father will not forgive your sins.

—Matthew 6:14–15 NIV

Then Peter came to Jesus and asked, "Lord, how many times shall I forgive my brother when he sins against me? Up to seven times?" Jesus answered, "I tell you, not seven times, but seventy-seven times."

—Matthew 18:21–22 NIV

If we confess our sins, he is faithful and just and will forgive us our sins and purify us from all unrighteousness.

—1 John 1:9 NIV

The LORD is merciful and gracious, slow to anger and abounding in steadfast love. He will not always chide, nor will he keep his anger forever. He does not deal with us according to our sins, nor repay us according to our iniquities. For as high as the heavens are above the earth, so great is his steadfast love toward those who fear him; as far as the east is from the west, so far does he remove our transgressions from us.

—Psalm 103:8–12 ESV

"…Come to me, all who labor and are heavy laden, and I will give you rest. Take my yoke upon you, and learn from me, for I am gentle and lowly in heart, and you will find rest for your souls. For my yoke is easy, and my burden is light."

—Matthew 11:28–30 ESV

Prayer

Dear God, thank You for not judging us using our standards. Thank You for being merciful and patient with us. Lord, thank You for sacrificing Your son Jesus for our undeserving souls. Lord, please give us guidance in exercising forgiveness. I ask that you make the recipients of our forgiveness and apologies receptive. Heavenly Father, please release us from the bondage of not forgiving. I pray that we are not only readers of the Word but that we apply Your Word to our everyday lives. These blessings I ask in the name of Jesus. Amen.

What do you need to forgive yourself for?

STRONG WOMEN ARE MISUNDERSTOOD

The LORD gives strength to his people; the LORD blesses his people with peace.

—*Psalm 29:11 NIV*

There are many strong women in the world, and, as one of them, I can truly say that strength can be both a blessing and a curse. Often, when one is viewed as a strong, independent woman, people believe she can handle everything. They view her as someone who doesn't need help. People will put more on her because they think of her as the go-to person to handle their issues. People may not consider the feelings of strong women because the theory is that "she can handle it."

What life experiences make a woman strong? In some cases, the presence of an adult may be lacking in the home, and a girl has to assume the role of an adult to keep the household running. Stepping into that role forces the girl to grow up faster and to become strong. Another scenario could be that the woman has experienced tragedy in her life, forcing her to take control of situations she normally wouldn't have to take on. Or consider the woman who doesn't feel she has anyone she can depend on for help in everyday life, and she becomes stronger day by day as she takes on the responsibility for everything.

Regardless of the reason that she becomes strong, we should always remember that the strong woman is human. As a strong woman, I must admit that I don't always want to be strong. Sometimes, I would rather not have so much responsibility in my life. I want someone to offer me a shoulder to lean on. It would be great if someone else made the major decisions sometimes. I would prefer not to be judged when I shed some tears or show a sign of weakness. As a strong woman, I am sometimes exhausted from taking care of everyone else and carrying the weight of so many people or things. Strong women sometimes feel alone.

I'm here to tell you that God wants you to seek Him in all that you do. Cast your cares upon the Lord, and wait patiently; He will give you rest. It's time to stop being Superwoman. Make a list of all your responsibilities and activities. Determine what is truly important, and evaluate what will happen if you no longer handle some of those responsibilities or perform those activities. Make an effort to remove three to five items from your list. Now consider replacing at least one of the items that you removed from the list with a pampering activity for yourself. It could be something as simple as driving to the beach to watch the sunset a few times per month or possibly getting a manicure, pedicure, or massage. You may want to consider just having a carefree lunch with a close friend or relative. Regardless, spend time just talking to God and meditating on Word. You must take care of yourself or you will no longer be equipped to help others.

Take it from me: Strong women are misunderstood. I am grateful for learning my strength from my mom and grandma. Strong women do have feelings, too. Strong women do experience hurt, disappointment, and a tremendous amount of stress. Women with strength need a shoulder to lean on from time to time. They need to be held and made to feel like they're loved. More than anything, they need to know from the actions of others in their lives that they have people to depend on in their times of need. One of the hardest things for a strong woman to do is ask for help. This is sometimes due to the mentality of "if you want something done right, you must do it yourself." It could also be because in the past when she has asked for help, she didn't receive it.

It took strength for me to share my life experiences in this book. I am usually pretty private about my past and my feelings. But as I started to recognize how much God has kept me through these experiences, I felt compelled to share my experiences and testimony with others. Pouring out my feelings has been like therapy for me. It has been a tremendous release of things, and I even literally feel like I have lost some weight after writing this. I had no intentions of hurting anyone by sharing my experiences my soul purpose is to give someone hope and comfort.

To my fellow strong women I say to you do not grow weary. Do not apologize for or boast about your strength. God's Word tells us to be strong. Do pray for the spirit of discernment. Discernment will tell you when to ask for help and who to ask for help. Continuously pray for restoration so that you can be replenished for all that you put out for others and so that you can continue to serve others. You need to understand that it is OK to say NO. The more you pray about discernment, you will receive guidance on what things you need to stay away from as well as what things you need to focus your time and talents on. So embrace your strength, be humble that God made you a strong woman, and get the rest necessary to go through this thing called life.

You will find great examples of strong women by reading the book of Ruth. Ruth and Naomi were both strong and courageous. Esther, Mary the mother of Jesus, Mary Magdalene, and Elizabeth the mother of John the Baptist. Learn about their values and character. Identify characteristics that you admire about these strong women in the bible and consider adopting and developing these skills for yourself.

Think twice the next time you see a strong woman. Instead of judging her or labeling her, ponder for a moment how and why she became so strong. Think of how you feel when you are labeled or even rejected. Think of how you feel when you are overwhelmed. Then decide if you still want to place that label on her or reject her.

The next time you encounter a strong woman, show her some compassion and respect. Consider giving her a hug. Offer to take over one of her responsibilities and actually complete it. Pray for her to receive rest, and pray that her strength is renewed day by day. Acknowledge that you know she has a lot on her plate, and offer her encouragement and prayer.

■ ■ ■

Wait for the LORD; be strong and take heart and wait for the LORD.

—Psalm 27:14 NIV

The God who equipped me with strength and made my way blameless. He made my feet like the feet of a deer and set me secure on the heights. He trains my hands for war, so that my arms can bend a bow of bronze.

—Psalm 18:32–34 ESV

The LORD is my strength and my song, and he has become my salvation; this is my God, and I will praise him, my father's God, and I will exalt him.

—Exodus 15:2 NIV

Seek the LORD and his strength; seek his presence continually!

—1 Chronicles 16:11 ESV

Prayer

Dear Lord, I pray for rest and renewed power and strength for the misunderstood strong women in the world. Lord, You know the desires of their hearts; please stand in the gap when they need help. May these women seek Your guidance in all that they say and do. Heavenly Father, please help others to understand them better and empathize with the demands on the lives of these women. Lord, I pray that these women do as Your Word says in Psalm 121 and look to the hills for help. These blessings I ask in the name of Jesus. Amen.

Are you a strong woman feeling misunderstood?

STEP INTO YOUR EXCELLENCE

For I know the plans I have for you, declares the LORD, plans for welfare and not for evil, to give you a future and a hope.

—*Jeremiah 29:11 NIV*

At some point all individuals will face obstacles, trials and tribulations in his/her life. We shouldn't expect to be exempt from these things after all even Jesus faced them. What I do know is *Philippians 3:13-14 NIV* says we should, "*Rejoice in the Lord always, I will say again: Rejoice!*"

Don't get stuck no matter what situation or circumstance you face in your life. People can learn a lot about a person by how they handle the storms in their life. This behavior shows you the character of an individual. Some will wallow in the circumstance or situation. While others will keep moving through it until it is over. Your mindset is very important and can influence how you react to a storm in your life. So if you choose to be a victim instead of a victor that will impact how you react in a storm. Don't run from challenges in life and when you have to fight always known that God is there with you in battle. You can't change your past but you can learn from it and build a better present and future. Don't get stuck, don't give up and believe that God has big plans for your life.

I have shared only a few of the trials and tribulations that I have faced in my life. Again, my reason for sharing is that my story may be a blessing to people going through similar situations. I pray that in some way those who are hurting can find comfort and strength in knowing that if God did all this for me, He can do that and more for them. God didn't create people to be miserable or to fail. God created us to be strong and to prosper. He created us to be compassionate and not depressed. He created us to love and not hate. But most importantly, God created us to be conquerors.

A relationship with God is personal. Only you can develop that relationship. While others can petition to God on our behalf, there is nothing like knowing and talking to God for yourself. Also, know that every conversation with God should not be your asking Him to do something for you. We should also talk to God and thank Him for things He has done, is doing, and will do in our lives. We should talk to God, repent, and ask for forgiveness for our sins.

I believe the enemy tends to attack those who are a threat, meaning that those who have a promising future and are blessed and favored will be on the front lines of attack. If you don't feel you are worthy of life, promotions, happiness, prosperity, and so forth, then no one else will feel you deserve it either. Always encourage yourself and seek God's Word for direction and encouragement in every situation. Also, be a blessing and encourage others. Let your light shine and walk in your purpose. Claim your blessings that God has stored up for you and you alone.

Habakkuk 2:2 reads, "Then the Lord replied write down the revelation and make it plain on tablets so that a herald may run with it." So I tell you, put your dream in writing. Start researching what it takes to achieve your dream. Seek God for guidance and favor. Find a person who is living your dream or something close to it. Reach out to them to learn what it will take for you to reach your dream. You may want to create a vision board and keep it where you can see it every day as a reminder of what you are working toward.

Set goals for your dream. Look up SMART goals; this will teach you how to establish goals. Actively work on your goals and celebrate your small successes, but keep on working until you achieve your dream. This will require a sacrifice of your time and money. It will require you to build up your skill set and to believe in your ability. There is no room for excuses. The only person you will let down is yourself. You must speak life over your dreams. You have probably heard that the only time that success comes before work is in the dictionary. So roll up your sleeves and put in that work.

Make the decision to work on your dream. Make the decision to invest in yourself as much as you invest in your favorite designer clothes, shoes, bags, and so forth. The same way you invest in a luxury vehicle. The same way you invest in brand name foods, vacations, makeup. Typically, we are quick to give away our money to purchase material things that make someone else wealthy. Meanwhile, we are apprehensive or will not invest in the training, coaching, or education required to help us achieve our own dreams.

Even if you feel that you are at your best now, please know that God can still make your life even better. You may find that hard to believe, but God is the ultimate giver. After all, He gave His only begotten son, giving us eternal life. Why not believe that God would do anything for you? Never think that your life is a mistake or that you are not worthy. Never give up on yourself because God will never give up on you. You definitely should never give up on God because He has your back and is working on your behalf even when we don't ask Him to. Keep the faith, and remember, you can be resilient on purpose!

According to the dictionary, *resilient* as it relates to a person means "the ability to withstand or recover quickly from difficult conditions." The definition of on *purpose* is intentionally or by intent. With all the trials and tribulations I have faced in my life so far, God has given me the ability to be resilient on purpose. God has delivered me from heartbreak and heartache, from sickness, from grief, and so many other things. God has unleashed a purpose in me for living my life to the fullest that is so strong, I can't contain it. I am excited about my future. I am grateful that God made obstacles in my life opportunities. I am thrilled to be a child of the Most High King.

Never apologize for the blessings you have received and will receive. Do share your blessings with others so they can see the mighty work of God. Don't block your blessings by being disobedient. God's instructions are always very specific. Step through the door that He opens. Don't question the doors that He closes. Wait patiently for your season of grace and favor. Do not become a victim of your past, a circumstance, or a situation. Trust, believe, and work faithfully. Listen for direction from God.

Luke 12:48 tells us that to whom much is given, much is required. God has already given us more than we would ever image. He made the ultimate sacrifice by giving His son, Jesus, to save us. So just think about that for a minute. With that in mind, we should always give our best in all situations. God requires us to be good stewards, to serve others, to love one another, to be witnesses, to show compassion, to take care of ourselves, and to be living examples of His grace and mercy. So I challenge you to step into your excellence and be passionate about the rest of your life. Don't be cocky, but do be confident because you are a child of God. Also, be humble in your journey.

Meditate on Psalm 91. It confirms that God has you covered at all times. Become passionate about your life because no one else will. Start living the life you love. Give yourself permission to be happy, to be great, and to be loved. Start laughing and laugh out loud. Laughter can be like medicine for your soul. Smile because it is infectious, and there is no harm in spreading joy.

■ ■ ■

For God gave us a spirit not of fear but of power and love and self-control.

—2 Timothy 1:7 ESV

No, in all these things we are more than conquerors through him who loved us.

—Romans 8:37 NIV

Have I not commanded you? Be strong and courageous. Do not be frightened, and do not be dismayed, for the Lord your God is with you wherever you go."

—Joshua 1:9 ESV

Whoever dwells in the shelter of the Most High will rest in the shadow of the Almighty. I will say of the Lord, "He is my refuge and my fortress, my God, in whom I trust."

—Psalm 91:1–2 NIV

Prayer

Dear God, I pray that this book is used to be a witness to unbelievers and to stir up hope in believers. I pray that my experiences show that by trusting and believing in You, all things are possible. Though bad things may come, we need to always pray without ceasing. I thank You, Lord, for the courage to write and share my stories. I pray that new relationships with God will be birthed as a result of reading this. I pray that existing relationships with God will be strengthened. I pray that someone is inspired to follow his or her dreams. I pray that estranged relationships between parents and children regardless of age are restored. I pray that we all become diligent in our forgiveness of others as well as ourselves. These blessings I ask in the name of Jesus. Amen.

Are you ready to step into your excellence?

Special Thanks

https://www.fiverr.com/maxphotomaster for my cover design
Macktography @macktographyinc for my cover photo
Jay Tee at Rated Pretty Girl Makeup Artistry for my makeup
Crystal at Honeyglobe Hair Salon for my hair

ABOUT SHINESE

"A woman who walks in purpose doesn't have to chase people or opportunities. Her light causes people and opportunities to pursue her." – Anne Nwakama

Shinese Collins is fiercely committed to guiding rising female leaders and executives to achieve career advancement by owning their careers, building powerful personal brands and building confidence to become a powerful presenter that will ultimately allow you to claim your success. If you are looking for a proven professional who can help you to address your fear of presenting, overcome your lack of confidence and to improve your image you've come to the right place.

Throughout her two decades in the telecommunications industry, Shinese has acquired extensive communication, relationship-building, planning, presentation, coaching, and development expertise. Founder and CEO of Powerful and Polished Presenters™ and Shinese Collins, LLC.

In addition, she has received several certifications, including Certified Life Coach (CLC), Certified Transformational Coach (CTC), and Certified Six Sigma Green Belt (CSSG). She also serves as the co-chair of the mentoring program for the Virginia Chapter of Women in Cable Telecommunications™.

Shinese is also a National Association of Professional Women 2016-2017 VIP Woman of the Year Circle Inductee. Personally she loves being a wife and a mother. To date, her number one passion is helping others transform their lives to achieve their dreams on both a professional and personal level. To learn more about Shinese visit www.shinesemcollins@cox.com .

Made in the USA
Columbia, SC
09 September 2022